Shame-Free ~ 2

Shame-Free

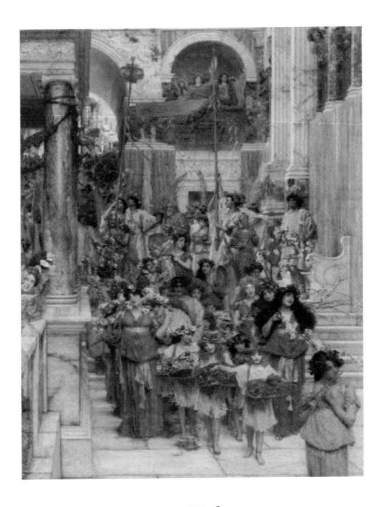

Jeanne Halsey

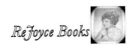
ReJoyce Books

Endorsements

Tremendously Touching Story

Jeanne has written a tremendously touching story that had me near tears more than once. I have no doubt that God can greatly use this book.

> ~ **Stanley Baldwin;** former pastor, best-selling author of *Love, Acceptance and Forgiveness* and *A Funny Thing Happened on My Way to Save Civilization.*

Source of Comfort

This story will be a source of comfort, particularly to Christian parents of unwed mothers. We, in the Church – who have received God's forgiveness and grace – tend to wrestle with guilt and shame far more than unbelievers do. Why is that? Having working in the Crisis Pregnancy Center Movement for over a dozen years, I remember many clients saying something like, "I'd rather face God with an abortion than the people at my church with an unplanned pregnancy." If only we understood how a judgmental attitude can actually be the gas that drives a young woman to an abortion clinic.

As Jeanne's family has discovered, God blesses when we made right choices. Sometimes it may take awhile for Him to work all things together for good, but as she so beautifully says, "When I could not sense 'hope' anywhere, at least I never lost that sense of His love for me. I held onto His love ... and He guided me through *'the valley of the shadow of shame'* (to paraphrase the Psalmist)."

> ~ **Julie Johnson;** former Director of Services at *Portland Pregnancy Resource Centers,* and a *Care Net* Medical Services Consultant (2003 through 2006)

An Attention-Getting Message

Psalm 45:1 speaks of *"the pen of a ready writer."* This phrase describes my daughter Jeanne most of her life. She has put volumes on paper to be a blessing to others. Under a large tent in Nairobi, Kenya, East Africa, I heard Jeanne share this subject *Shame-Free* in a service for women. It was an attention-getting message, one so many mothers there could relate to. Jeanne and her husband Ken handled this crisis in their lives with compassion and forgiveness. May this same message impact you like it did those hundreds of African women.

> ~ **Dr. Don Gossett;** 60-years as missionary-evangelist, author of best-selling *What You Say Is What You Get*, father of Jeanne Halsey

A Loving and Steady Hand

Jeanne Halsey's long-awaited book *Shame-Free* is a loving and steady hand guiding us through the mine-fields of Life's unexpected war zones. Her wisdom nuggets, gleaned from the trenches of conflict, whisper hope in the midst of midnight. She has journeyed through the obstacles and offers invaluable and practical strategies to not simply survive, but actually become strengthened through the process of forgiveness and tough love.

Shame-Free will be a "go-to" book for my staff and me as we counsel those overwhelmed by sudden shame.

> ~ **Dr. Reba Rambo-McGuire;** award-winning singer, author of *Follow the Yellow Brick Road*, pastor of *The River at Music City* Church in Nashville, Tennessee

Shame-Free
By Jeanne Halsey

ISBN 978-0-557-41181-81-8

For more information, contact:

ReJoyce Books

4424 Castlerock Drive

Blaine, Washington 98230

United of America

www.halseywrite.com

Table of Contents

Dedication

There are three entities responsible for this book. First are the wonderful staff of the *Whatcom County Pregnancy Clinic,* especially **Nancy Fischer,** a volunteer counselor, and my dear friend **Carol Thomas,** the former Executive Director of the Clinic.

One day while I was visiting the staff at the Clinic, Nancy rather innocently asked me if I knew of any books or materials that would help shocked and grieving parents who have just learned their teenage daughter (or son) is pregnant, outside of marriage. When my husband Kenneth and I were first going through the deep sorrow of our beautiful daughter Jennifer admitting her unplanned pregnancy at age 16, caring friends from our church had lent us different books designed to help us ... but as the years passed, I honestly did not remember the titles or authors of any of those books. I had long since returned them to their original owners, or had lent them to other parents in similar straits. In that casual conversation with Nancy – who had just that day been counseling parents whose teenage child's pregnancy test was positive – I was quite suddenly reminded by God I had written *this* book so many years ago (now out-of-print). When I also realized there is a whole new chapter to follow-up, I was energized to rewrite the book ... which you are reading today.

It was my great privilege to serve on the Board of Directors of the Whatcom County Pregnancy Clinic, to be a small part of the great work they are doing to help save lives – the lives of the unborn, and the lives of parents who are faced with an unplanned pregnancy. We have a far greater percentage of clients who choose life rather than abortion ... and for that, we give God all the glory.

I dedicate this book to the Clinic, believing that God will continue to use this ministry with power and the result of saving lives ... and I particularly honor Carol Thomas for her 15 years of dedication to a very difficult ministry, at which she excelled.

The second person responsible for this book is our wonderful first grandson, **Kristian Michael Alexander Freeman** – he who 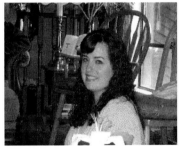 was that "unplanned" baby. I joyfully dedicate this book to him because he has so marvelously changed our lives. In the 17 years since I wrote the first version, Kristian has grown into an incredible young man, brilliant, charming, handsome, very, very tall ... and continually a bright light for Christ Jesus. If it had not been for him, this book would never have been written. Every day I thank God for Kristian.

Lastly, I dedicate this book to our precious daughter **Jennifer Elisabeth Joy (Halsey) Freeman,** whom I have always loved from the bottom of my heart and beyond. Our journey through life has not always been easy, but she is totally worth it to us. Because of her, we have been enriched beyond measure. *"Thank you, Jennifer, for being ... and thank You, Heavenly Father, for giving her to us."*

Jeanne "Grammy" Halsey

Blaine, Washington ~ April 2010

Foreword

By **Anne Ryan**

"This is like seeing an open wound from a dagger to the heart."

That is what I remember thinking when I saw Jeanne and Kenneth after they had learned their 16-year-old daughter was pregnant out-of-wedlock. Then fear wafted over me as we are the parents of four girls: *"These are good parents – no, great parents! – with a very loving supportive extended family who loves the Lord and serves Him. They have raised their kids in the church in fact, in our church. If they couldn't avoid this, then who can successfully guide their children through this stormy time of life?"* And this was not the only family in our church to negotiate this pain.

My husband is their pastor, and our son is best friends with their son. Jeanne and I have been in Bible Studies together. Kenneth has led our Worship teams. Their pain was our pain, and yet I am sure they felt confused, alone ... and ashamed.

If you have picked up this book because your family is facing a similar situation, then perhaps it will help you to process your pain, heal and be released from shame. Jeanne has turned to our loving Heavenly Father and processed the healing of that opened wound. She didn't just let skin grow over so it doesn't look so bad – she really reached deep into the layers of her heart, and let God heal her.

This story has a wonderful ending. Perhaps your story won't end as well, but this I know: if you let the Lord into your story, the ending will be much better than if you don't. May the God of all comfort, the Lord of all mercy, heal you to the point of being *shame-free!*

Longtime friend Anne Ryan is the wife of Dr. Kim Ryan, Jeanne and Kenneth's pastor at North County Christ the King Community Church, in Lynden, Washington. Anne is formerly a Board Member of the Whatcom County Pregnancy Clinic.

Introduction

Perhaps the most often asked question of Modern Man is: *"Why do bad things happen to good people?"*

Depending on circumstances, getting to the bottom of that query may take forever, or may never be answered at all. This is my story ... and I'm going to start with a **SPOILER ALERT: this story has a happy ending!** To be honest, when I wrote the first version of this book in 1994, I was in a very sad place – heartbroken, struggling to understand, deeply concerned about our daughter and her child, uncertain of their future. When I was in turmoil, I did what I have always done: I journaled, and from that journal I eventually published the first version of *Shame-Free*. It was meant to help others who have found themselves in this same (or similar) scenario to know that God still cares about them ... because I had discovered that He still cared about me!

Another hallmark of my struggle through shame was that the original version utilized changed names and modified situations, because I didn't really want to admit to the world that I was writing my own story – which, in itself, was a measure of the impact of my shame. In rewriting and updating this book, I have totally dumped all those disguised references and am now telling this story in real-time, with real identities revealed. This authentic version is a true measure of the healing which God worked in my heart, showing how thoroughly He has cleansed me from shame.

This is my own very subjective story; others may remember it differently than I. Also, I cannot begin to address every situation – such as a pregnant child who comes from a single-parent home ... an unexpected pregnancy the result of rape or incest ... a pregnant child who is addicted to substance abuse – but there is one truth **everyone** can hold onto: **God can work deeply in your heart and lift you out of the dead-end weight of shame in your life.** It takes hope ... and patience ... and trust that He knows better than you about the outcome of your life.

I sought the Lord, and He answered me; He delivered me from all my fears. Those who look to Him are radiant; their faces are never covered with shame.

Psalm 34:4-5

Part One: **Colossians 2:15**

For I want you to know what a great conflict I have for you ... that your hearts may be encouraged, being knit together in love, and attaining to all riches of the full assurance of understanding to the knowledge of the mystery of God, both of the Father and of Christ. ... As you therefore have received Christ Jesus the Lord, so walk in Him rooted and built up in Him, and established in the faith as you have been taught, abounding in it with thanksgiving. ... And you are complete in Him, Who is the Head of all principality and power.

As you have therefore received Christ, even Jesus the Lord, so walk (regulate your lives and conduct yourselves) in union with and conformity to Him. Have the roots of your being firmly and deeply planted [in Him, fixed and founded in Him], being continually built up in Him, becoming increasingly more confirmed and established in the faith, just as you have been taught, and abounding and overflowing in it with thanksgiving. ...

*And you, being dead in your trespasses ... **He has made alive together with Him, having forgiven you all trespasses ... He has taken it out of the way, having nailed it to the cross. Having disarmed principalities and powers, He made a public spectacle of them, triumphing over them.***

Colossians 2:1-3, 6-7, 9-10, 13-15 (emphasis added)

Chapter 1: **"It Will Never Happen to Us"**

It was quite warm under the canvas overhang on that African afternoon, but that wasn't why I was perspiring. I was nervous because there were probably 500 women of all ages, waiting to hear me speak ... and the prepared comments I had in hand were just about to be proverbially tossed out the window.

This was a special Ladies Meeting at the Nairobi Pentecostal Church, South Campus, in Kenya, East Africa, and I had accompanied my father, Rev. Don Gossett, on a missions trip to one of my favorite African nations. The pastors, Dennis and Esther White, were family friends I had known since my teen years. Now that I was all grown up, I was honored by their request to speak to their ladies. I had written out notes about some encouraging topic – but suddenly I was hearing a Voice inside telling me to speak about something entirely different. It was the Voice I have learned to obey.

"A few years ago," I began, "Dad and I went on a missions trip to Australia, and on the day when I returned home, nearly the first thing my 16-year-old daughter said to me was, 'Mom, I'm pregnant.'" I paused, gulping somewhat, and the room was completely silent. The women – teenage girls, mothers, grandmothers – were riveted on what I would say next.

"This is not something that usually happens in Christian families, or so I thought," I continued. "The impact on me and our entire family was world-shattering. It was the worst day of my whole life." As I continued responding to the urging of Holy Spirit, I sensed these words were hitting home with devastating reality, but also with a promise of hope and healing. By the end of the meeting, the result was an outpouring of honesty, sincere repentance, healing of broken relationships, and a renewed commitment to purity among the women.

Revealing this painful episode in my life was not really something I was eager to do, but being obedient to God's Voice was far more important than any personal discomfort I may have felt. The ability to share freely about my teenage daughter's pregnancy also represented a significant healing that had taken place in my own heart: I had been set free from shame! This true story is how it happened.

The Sermon on Shame

Have you ever sat through a great sermon at church but thought to yourself, "Well, that was great, but it doesn't really apply to me"? Early in 1990, a member of our church who is also a professional psychologist and counselor, Dr. David Anderson, shared a brief sermon series entitled something like "Overcoming Shame." He based it primarily on the great passage from Colossians 2:15, where the Apostle Paul wrote about the wonderful redemptive work of Jesus Christ on the cross:

And having spoiled principalities and powers, Christ made a show of them openly, triumphing over them in His crucifixion.

Or, as Dave eloquently stated it: ***"Jesus Christ put shame to shame."*** He described how, in the ancient Roman culture, when an army returned from battle to Rome, there would be a great parade when all the spoils of war – the loot, the treasures, and often the imprisoned enemies themselves – were triumphantly displayed before the whole populace, garnering more accolades for the soldiers and further dishonoring their enemies. Then the ultimate humiliation was carried out on most of the prisoners (those not chosen to be slaves): they were crucified in public.

Dave explained that in his work as a psychologist, many of his patients suffered from issues rooted in long-term shame – whether from situations they had allowed into their lives, or perhaps something from their childhood or family heritage. He shared how much of his counseling ministry included helping his patients accept complete forgiveness through Christ for their sins and learn how to erase debilitating shame from their lives.

Most emphatically, Dave talked about this verse, which he interpreted this way: "When we accept God's forgiveness for sins in our lives, Christ Himself becomes our Victor, and He nails our sins to His own cross, forever removing their effects from our lives. Then He holds a parade, or a show, of those defeated sins and shame, and those situations which once had so impacted our lives negatively are now held up as trophies of His defeat over their power in our lives." The sentence I remember most from his sermon was: *"Christ Jesus put Shame to shame."*

While Dave's sermons were great and memorable, I honestly did not think they applied to my life. I just stowed them away somewhere in the back of my mind, never knowing how important those principles would very soon become to me.

Our Little Family

Kenneth Halsey and I were married in May 1974, when he was 22 and I was 20. He came from a family with three older sisters; I had an older brother, an older sister, a younger brother, and a younger sister. "Family" was something we both appreciated, and we were happy when God blessed our family with two lovely children: Jennifer Elisabeth Joy (born November 1975, when I was 22), and Alexander John Edward (born January 1978; I was 24).

Since there is really no true preparation for parenting except the actual experience itself, Kenneth and I were uncertain about our skills as parents, but our hearts were wide-open to the task. Of course, we talked with our contemporaries and watched their parenting, but we knew we needed to rely strongly on God's grace and presence to walk us through our process.

Kenneth was beside me for the birth of Jennifer, and I recall the overwhelming love and joy we experienced when we first looked into her astonishingly intelligent eyes and met this wonderful child who was absolutely ours! And Jennifer was the most beautiful baby ever born (I have tons of photographs in proof), and she totally delighted our entire extended family, especially since she was the first grandchild on my side of the family. People often commented on her appearance: her abundant dark hair, fair skin, green eyes, petite figure, and her vivacious, sweet personality. Kenneth and I felt amazingly blessed to have such a perfect daughter.

The Other Child

There was, however, an interesting event which took place shortly after Jennifer was born. I had breastfed her from birth, so I was not surprised when my normal menstrual cycle had not resumed by the time I took her for her regular five-month checkup. After examining Jennifer thoroughly and pronouncing her healthy, our family doctor additionally remarked, "Jeanne, you look unusually pale to me. Let's do urine and blood tests." (The only glitch experienced during my pregnancy with Jennifer had been a tendency toward anemia; I was given iron shots several times to boost red blood cells.)

It was shocking when I received a phone call from the doctor the next day: I was at least two months pregnant! Dr. Wong said, "You need to come back for the prenatal exam." His further examination confirmed this pregnancy, and he added, "Since you cannot nourish three people at the same time (yourself, Jennifer, and the fetus), you need to stop nursing your baby." When I shared this news with Kenneth, he was also stunned; this meant we had conceived again when Jennifer was three months old, and we would have two children exactly one year apart! In truth, it took us several days to process and accept the fact that we were going to again become parents very soon. Although she adapted to the bottle very easily, it was heartbreaking for me to wean my precious Jennifer from breast-milk.

Then – three or four weeks after the medical examination confirming pregnancy – just when we were reconciled to having another baby so soon and were now happily anticipating this new child, I began to experience very painful cramps. Within a few hours, I miscarried the baby. We were deeply sorrowful and grieved our lost child, and we began to carefully plan when our next child should be conceived. Two years and three months after Jennifer's birth, our wonderful son Alexander was born. We were consumed with joy at our beautiful little family. Jennifer totally claimed her brother as her own, and they developed a sweet sibling relationship.

There is another aspect about this miscarried child – and you can choose if you believe this as I have no Biblical proof to confirm this. I have always been a vivid dreamer, and could usually remember my night's dreams in great detail the next morning. It can't truly be called a prophetic gift, but often aspects of my dreams came to pass later. In 1992, I had an extremely clear dream which has brought immeasurable comfort to me.

In this dream, my sweet mother Joyce Gossett (who had prematurely died of heart disease in August 1991) was happily working away in the most glorious garden imaginable (gardening was her passion). I was walking toward her along a heavenly arboreal pathway. Working with Mom was a tall young man, and as I approached, they both stood up to greet me.

I was so happy to see my beloved mother again, but I was puzzled by her coworker. After I joyfully embraced Mom, I turned to the young man with question in my eyes. "Don't you know who this is, Jeanne?" Mom asked. She then clarified, "Jeanne, this is your son. This is David, the baby you miscarried." Our child was **not** a little infant – he was a full-grown, handsome adult! He had a name, he had a purpose, he had an active relationship with his grandmother. He *is* alive and well in Heaven.

Since then, I have repeatedly dreamed about David, who was usually doing something ordinary with my mother, or with my sister Judy Gossett (who tragically died of cancer in 2003). I believe God gives me these dreams or visions of the child we lost to miscarriage. I genuinely anticipate meeting him one day.

Multiplication

We so adored Jennifer! She was the perfect baby: enchanting, beautiful, personable, charming to everyone. People were always remarking on her outstanding looks and sweet personality. Often total strangers would comment, "What a gorgeous child!"

When Jennifer celebrated her second birthday, Kenneth, Jennifer and I accompanied my father and mother on a trip to Florida. Before each departure-leg, little Jennifer stood up in the aisle seat of the airplane and personally greeted every passenger, to their obvious delight. Another time, Kenneth and I went out of town and left our two young children in the care of my parents. When Jennifer and Alexander were riding in the car with their grandparents, they became a little too boisterous for the adults and so were scolded by my father. Jennifer piped up, "Grandpa, when I come to your house, I don't come to be yelled at." She enchanted everyone.

For a first-time mother, I couldn't have asked for a better experience. Jennifer was "by the book" at teething, sitting up, learning to talk, but she jumped ahead by walking proficiently at 9 months and showing superior physical motor skills. She was not, however, so good at sleeping because she seemed wired to require less sleep than "normal" – there were many early morning awakenings by this beautiful baby standing right next to our bed, smiling angelically into our sleepy faces. Many,

many times we simply thanked God for giving us such an incredible child.

      While I was pregnant with Alexander, I recall having mixed feelings about adding another child to our family. These feelings had to do with naively wondering how in the world I would be able to love another child half as much as I loved Jennifer. It was then God taught me His principle of multiplication: my heart was not going to be divided between our children – He is the Maker of all things, and His plan is multiplication, not division. He simply expanded my heart to love **more,** not to have less love to share.

Chapter 2: **In the "Best" of Families**

In the 1970s, the "ideal" North American family consisted of two parents and 2.3 children (just how do you get that fraction of a child?), and we were strongly counseled – I would even say coerced – to "conclude" our family with our one girl and one boy. Kenneth underwent a vasectomy, which I later realized was a big mistake because my heart really hungered for more children. I had two brothers and two sisters, while Kenneth had three sisters and no brothers – and I wanted my children to each be able to experience the joy of having at least one same-gender sibling. However, the vasectomy was final, and so we concentrated on loving and enjoying the two wonderful children God had given us.

Being Raised In (and Raising) a Christian Family

Growing up in the household of a traveling Christian evangelist, it was built into my cells that we – meaning the five children, of whom I was third in line – should never, ever do anything to disgrace our parents. There was some "higher standard" that PKs (preacher's kids) were required to maintain ... and throughout my childhood and teen years, if ever I was tempted to transgress – cheat on a school test, use bad language, steal a package of gum from the corner store – there was this built-in restrictor that kept me "straight and narrow."

Never in my wildest dreams would I willingly get involved with anything like premarital sex, or alcohol, or any form of criminal activity. Those behaviors were against my parents' teachings; more importantly, they were against God's Law. I was not perfect, but it was deep in my hear that I never wanted to do anything that would bring shame to my family, nor to the Name of my Savior and Lord Jesus Christ.

Kenneth, like me, was born into a Christian family, and he grew up with well-defined rules and regulations of living as a Christian. We both were taught there was a "scale" of sins that ranged from "not so bad" to "really dangerous." Among the "big ones" were those concerning sex outside of marriage, and the consequences that could result from promiscuity.

We reared our children, to have successful lives, that they should honor God in everything. We educated Jennifer and Alexander about right and wrong, good and evil, the rewards of good choices and the challenges of bad choices. This included openly discussing the Godly place of sex within marriage, and aspects of healthy sexuality. We emphasized the consequences of sexual activity outside of marriage, which is so prevalent in our sex-saturated culture – everything from sexually transmitted diseases, to homosexuality, to unplanned pregnancy and the evils of abortion. We raised Jennifer and Alexander in the same home, at the same time, with the same principles ... and we believed because they were both born-again believers in Jesus Christ, they would each make good Christian decisions with their lives at the right time.

Jennifer was (and is) very pretty, very bright, very personable, and very self-assured. Without excessive parental pressure, she excelled in academics, worked diligently to maintain high grades, was a popular cheerleader (the result of many years of gymnastic lessons), was a member of the school's student council, had a wide circle of friends, and was faithful to attend church with us. She had strong goals for her life, a plan to use her talents in TV programming, perhaps as a broadcast producer or journalist. Kenneth and I were very proud of our "perfect princess," and we trusted her completely.

Kenneth especially has a warm, loving relationship with our daughter. She is much more like him in temperament and character, while Alexander is more like me. There was never a trace of the classic "searching for a father-figure" element that often plagues troubled teenage girls.

When it came to teaching our children about purity, Kenneth had a funny little saying which he often repeated to Jennifer: "Honey, there's just one thing that boys want ... and you don't want to give it to them." He exhorted this mantra so often, it became the family joke. Jennifer knew it was true, and as she matured into a beautiful teenager, it was evident she was very capable of holding the boys at bay. Young men flocked to Jennifer, and she had a following of handsome boys who would do her every bidding just because they adored her ... and while she didn't actually encourage them, she knew how to control them.

The Conspiracy of Silence

Early in 1992, there was a conversation which I recall very clearly. Kenneth was away on a business trip, so it was only Jennifer, Alexander and I at home eating dinner. That day we had learned one of Jennifer's classmates, Karen, was pregnant; she was only 15 years old. I recall the sorrow and pity I felt for Karen's parents, and my dismay for her future. As we thoughtfully discussed this situation, Jennifer asked me very seriously, "Mom, what would you do if you found out I was pregnant?"

I struggled to formulate an answer. "Honey, if that happened, I would be shocked! It would be so painful. I just can't imagine what it would be like to have a 15-year-old daughter get pregnant." Then I looked very deeply into her brilliant green eyes. "Jennifer, you aren't sexually active, are you?" Of course, she immediately denied that, reassuring me she was only asking a rhetorical question. Inwardly, I sighed with relief, because I believed her. We so totally trusted our daughter.

The conversation then turned to the impression that "nearly everyone" in our little town already knew about Karen's situation. There is this maddening concept rampant among teens which I call the "conspiracy of silence." For months,

Jennifer and her contemporaries had known Karen and her boyfriend were sexually active; therefore it really didn't come as a shock to most that she was now pregnant. I despaired of this "conspiracy of silence" code because I believe that if just one person, just one true friend, just one caring individual might have spoken up and asked Karen and her boyfriend, "Don't you know the perils of premarital sex? Don't you know the risks of unprotected sex?" – perhaps her predicament might have been avoided.

Then the Lord asked Cain, "Where is Abel your brother?"

Cain replied, "I do not know. Am I my brother's keeper?"

Genesis 4:9

The fact is: kids think they're doing their friends a favor by concealing their illicit activities. Around this same time, there was an incident where a popular young boy in school somehow acquired someone else's credit cards, and he went on a spending spree, buying expensive clothes and electronics for his friends. Eventually he was caught, and he ended up spending years in Juvenile Detention. None of his friends thought it wise to report his illegal use of stolen credit cards – and none of them had to return the expensive things he had so generously bought for them. How different that boy's life would have been if just one person among the many who knew about the stolen credit cards would have called a halt before it became serious! In my opinion, as unpopular as it may seem, it is wrong to stay silent.

Shortly after this memorable conversation, we learned Karen's boyfriend had dumped her, and his family disavowed the pregnancy and any further responsibility he would carry. In fact, they urged Karen to give up the baby for adoption, but she and her parents decided against that. Several months later, Karen gave birth to a daughter, whom she decided to keep and raise alone, despite the boyfriend's objections.

I recall sometimes seeing Karen's mother at the grocery store, her infant granddaughter riding in the shopping basket while her daughter was at school. She said having a baby at home again since so many years had passed from raising their own children was a challenge, but the baby was loved and that was what mattered. I agreed with her, sympathetic ... but inwardly grateful we were spared this scenario in our lives.

The truth is: within the next few years, three more of Jennifer's schoolmates – and even three of her own biological cousins! – would become pregnant out-of-wedlock. Teenage sex is a sorry fact of life in our society, and the shocking consequences don't seem to matter that much to them:

In 1995, there were over 500,000 births to teenagers, over 200,000 to those not even 18 years of age. The teenage population is growing, and if teenage birth rates do not continue to decline, there will be a rise in the number of teenage births over the next few years. ... Non-marital births totaled just over 1.2-million in 1995, and accounted for 31-percent of all births that year.

— **Center for Disease Control**

Chapter 3: **The Day and Night of Shock**

We loved and trusted our "perfect" daughter – we did **not** know Jennifer was actually leading a double-life. In her early teens, she became adept at sneaking out of her bedroom window in the middle of the night, and joining her friends for illicit fun-and-games. We had no idea at all she was hanging out with other underage kids who were drinking and taking drugs, although neither alcohol or drugs had any attraction to her. Jennifer quickly became the "designated driver" among her friends. And Jennifer was very curious about sex.

In retrospect, Kenneth and I wondered how this double-life had ever developed, what "chink" in Jennifer's personality might have attracted her to the "other side" ... and there was only one thing we could postulate. When Jennifer was 9 years old, Kenneth's employer transferred us to Dallas, Texas, and we transported our family halfway across the country, from the West Coast to the Southwest. We moved away from very close-knit family relationships which Jennifer had – especially with my youngest sister Marisa – and away from her school friends. All the way on our drive from Washington State to Texas, Jennifer wept ... and frequently vomited (not so much from carsickness, but from anguish). When we arrived at our new home in Texas, she was sullen and unhappy for weeks, until she finally began to make new friends at her new school.

We had frequents visits from our family back home, and we were able to take regular flights back to visit them too. Our mistake was believing that Jennifer trusted her parents enough to take in stride this upheaval in her life. Instead, she harbored deep disappointment, often acting angry with us, and we did not know how to help her as she changed so dramatically from the loving, vivacious child she had been. It was more than just adolescence – it was like she had a youthful nervous breakdown. We now presume her excessive sorrow led to a break in the protective armor we believed was there by God's grace.

When Kenneth's company eventually transferred us back to Washington State in the same year Jennifer entered high school, she found many of her friends from elementary school were still in town, and she quickly reconnected with them. It was with these old friends that she began to act out her double-life.

Pretty and personable Jennifer attracted many boys, as previously explained. She had a series of casual boyfriends who usually liked her a whole lot more than she liked them; it was just too easy for her to wrap any one of them around her little finger. Then she met Patrick Freeman. Patrick was two years older than her, two grades ahead of her in the same school. Patrick is a good-looking, self-possessed guy, and at first he viewed Jennifer as this bubbly, self-absorbed girl who was cute but not his type. However, since "opposites tend to attract," eventually they started dating. When I first met Patrick, I was amused that it seemed Jennifer had finally found a boyfriend she could **not** wrap around her finger!

The first years they dated, Jennifer and Patrick had an on-again, off-again relationship. They were often adversarial, and when they broke up, it usually resulted in many tears and hard feelings (at least witnessed on Jennifer's part). Kenneth and I never thought their relationship had any longevity, primarily because there was one critical aspect about Patrick that, to us, meant they would never be serious: Patrick was not a Christian. We specifically taught our children that it was always a mistake for a believer to marry a nonbeliever – or, as my father taught, "When a Christian marries a non-Christian, they will always have trouble with their 'father-in-law'" meaning Satan (*"How can two walk together except they be agreed?"* Amos 3:3).

The Truth Comes Out

In the spring of 1992, I accompanied my father on a four-week missions trip to Australia. One day while strolling through the beautiful Outback, Dad rhetorically asked me to "describe my two children to him" (he has always been a very fond grandfather, but he wanted to bask in my own estimation of Jennifer and Alexander). I spoke with pride about what wonderful kids God had given to Kenneth and me: both excelling academically, active in sports and extra-curricular activities, leaders in school with student body positions, faith-filled and enthusiastic at church. Dad and I shared about an hour of happy memories of these, his two eldest grandchildren, and how they had wonderfully impacted the lives of all our extended family.

When I returned from that visit to Australia on a Friday in June 1992, my family warmly welcomed me home, with several members of our extended family lingering at our house to catch up. I happily distributed assorted gifts and souvenirs, related glowingly about the ministry in which I had helped Dad, and entertaining them with stories of kangaroos, koala bears and crocodiles. We all had a great visit after my long absence.

While the impromptu "welcome home party" was still going on, Jennifer asked me to come alone to her bedroom. She quietly closed the door. Then, very tentatively, she said, "Mom, I'm pregnant. I found out the week you left for Australia." For over a month, my 16-year-old daughter had known she was pregnant, but she was terrified to tell her father alone.

This news devastated me, and I fell down on her bed. I questioned her closely, verifying dates ... and asking her, "Oh, honey, has how this happened?" We both wept as she finally admitted she and Patrick had been intimate for over a year (she gave him her virginity). She had previously been taking birth-control pills (shockingly, a prescription she obtained without our knowledge or consent), but when they broke up (numerously), she stopped taking contraceptives. Then they started dating again, and eventually resumed sexual intercourse ... and she became pregnant.

Our visitors finally departed, and I called Kenneth into Jennifer's bedroom – and I am certain one of the hardest experiences in her entire life was telling her father this earth-shattering news. We both felt like our wonderful world with two perfect children had opened up beneath our feet and crashed all around us. We called in 14-year-old Alexander and told him too ... and our whole family wept together.

For the next several hours, we talked. And wept. And talked and wept. We are a very analytical family, but it was difficult to ferret out the pieces of this appalling puzzle and finally put together the picture of a daughter who smiled at us on the outside but who led a hidden, different life, unknown to us. Jennifer admitted the deep hurt she felt when our family moved to Texas had caused her to stop trusting her parents – an attitude for which she eventually repented.

Alexander confessed he knew a little about Jennifer's nighttime escapades, but he did not know how intimately involved she was with Patrick. We asked her, "Jennifer, why did you ever become sexually active?" Her answers were vague: "I was curious" ... "Well, I really love Patrick!" ... and "Everybody's doing it." She was correct about that last one:

Prior to 1993, there had been a 30-year rise in childbearing by unmarried women, and from 1980 to 1991, the rate increased 54-percent.

– U.S. Department of Health and Human Services

As we struggled to absorb this huge trauma, one thing was immediately apparent to me: it was critically important that Jennifer know we would never reject her ... or her child. Our emotions ran high – with Jennifer suggesting perhaps she should go stay at a friend's house – but I adamantly refused to let her go. I felt like Satan would achieve some kind of victory if she went outside the umbrella of our parental protection. I insisted she stay, that we had to work this out.

Immediately, Kenneth and I felt like total failures as parents. We had not even recognized any signs that our daughter had forsaken so much of her Christian heritage, and could successfully lead a double-life right under our noses. Now our precious, beautiful, beloved daughter had become a dreaded statistic: **an unmarried pregnant teenager.** As we slowly began to grasp the situation, Kenneth and I wrestled with: "Where did we go wrong?" ... "What past sins of our own have come back to haunt us now?" ... and "What generational curses are in our family that this would happen?"

Right away, we were faced with a huge dilemma: how were we going to tell our family and friends? This was totally uncharted territory for us, and a crushing fear of revealing the truth began to weigh on us. This was the beginning of the shame. We were broken people.

Chapter 4: **Terrible Options**

Immediately we decided we should take Jennifer to our family doctor, to see if possibly the at-home pregnancy tests might have been erroneous. I suppose all parents who see their children go astray always hope somehow it is a mistake, somehow it is not really the way it appears. Once the pregnancy was officially confirmed, however, we would talk about Jennifer's (and Patrick's) options, which eventually came down to these:

(1) Jennifer could have an abortion.

(2) She and Patrick could get married, and raise the baby together.

(3) She would have the baby, but then give him up for adoption.

(4) She and Patrick would not get married, but still raise the baby together (not living together).

Yes, even a Christian needs to talk about that terrible first option, because – God help us! – abortion is legal in the United States. In our state of Washington, an underage child can legally be prescribed contraceptives **without parental knowledge or consent**. Worse, *an underage child can legally have an abortion without parental knowledge or consent.* As much as we decried that option, we still knew abortion was one option our underage daughter could legally consider ... and it was ultimately her choice to make. We do not support abortion and spoke urgently against it, but tragically it **was** a legal, realistic choice on the list.

I believe life begins at conception, and I consider a child lost to abortion to be the same as a child lost to miscarriage. As

I previously related, I expect one day to meet in Heaven our miscarried child, our son David ... and I believe a parent who aborts her baby will also meet her child in Heaven. However, I do not believe an aborted child will blame or judge his parents for causing his death – judgment is God's business, not ours.

Kenneth and I also strongly urged Jennifer not to choose option two (marriage) either, for two very good reasons. First, she was only 16, Patrick was only 18 ... and they were simply too young to get married. The chances of being able to establish a healthy marriage with such high odds stacked against them were very slim. Being married – and staying married – is such a daunting task for anyone, Christian or otherwise ... and for them to get married because "they had to" did not bode well for a successful marriage. Second, and equally important to us, was the fact that Patrick was not a Christian, and we believed the teaching that states a Christian should not marry a non-Christian. Despite her "other lifestyle," Jennifer was still a practicing Christian.

Option three (adoption) was heart-rending, especially for me. While we realize there are many hopeful couples longing to adopt a child – my own brother and his wife, unable to have biological children, have happily adopted two beautiful kids – it just seemed impossible to imagine. I struggled with the concept that this child of our daughter's flesh and descended from ours, this tiny person already moving around inside her body, might go to live with some other family, no matter how wonderful they might be; and we would never know him or anything about him. This I could not bear. Having lost my mother to heart disease just one year before this crisis (at the young age of 62), the idea that an offspring of Joyce Gossett might never know his biological identity or anything about his spiritual heritage was too impossible to contemplate.

(My "other sister" Reba Rambo-McGuire knew of a wonderful Christian adoption agency, and she offered to fly Jennifer and me to check out this place in Tennessee.

However, although we do not deny the adoption choice, we knew it was not for Jennifer.)

Which left option four: that she would keep the baby and raise him herself, with some assistance from Patrick. This was the only option we could wholly endorse, but we also knew it carried a huge, huge cost – not so much financially (although that was very real) but in what it meant in the death of her dreams, her plans for her future, now totally shattered.

After a long, long evening of painful discussion, we finally went to bed. I am grateful our headstrong daughter elected **not** to leave our home that night, but retired to her own bedroom (window firmly locked!). It was so important to me to keep our family whole, and letting her leave – or from her perspective, she thought it might be best if she went to a friend's house for just one night – seemed to be an even bigger mistake.

God Shows Up

Kenneth and I lay in our bed, unable to sleep, staring up at the dark ceiling, hearts broken, reeling from shock, no clear path in sight. It was probably 2 or 3 in the morning, and we had cried our eyes dry, but still were sleepless and now speechless. Then into our bedroom walked our 14-year-old son Alexander ... and he made a simple statement that I believed then – and still believe today – was the voice of God's Holy Spirit speaking directly to us.

"Dad, Mom, you need to know something. You have been great parents. You have taught us right and wrong. You've done everything you could to help her make good decisions. *This was Jen's choice.* She's not stupid, she knew better, you taught us better, but she made a bad decisions, and these are her consequences, not yours. This is not your fault. This is Jen's choice."

With that, he turned and walked back to his own bedroom ... and somehow our eyes found even more tears to shed. However, for the first time since Jennifer had called me into her bedroom in the afternoon, I began to sense just the tiniest flicker of hope. We were overwhelmed with shock, sorrow and shame, searching for some understanding of how this could have occurred. *"In what area did we fail our daughter? At what point did we become oblivious to her real self?"* Perhaps more subtle, *"What did we do wrong ourselves that we must now pay this price in our daughter's life?"* When Alexander made his simple statement, for the first time we could entertain that perhaps we had not failed as parents ... and we could find strength to help Jennifer make good decisions in the days to come.

The following Saturday afternoon, we met with our pastor and shared our sad news. We offered to step off all positions of church leadership because we felt like we no longer deserved their trust or had proven ourselves to be "in control of our household." Our pastor and the church council graciously declined our offer. Instead, the church leadership and our "small group" surrounded us with love and support, which truly sustained us through the coming months. Our pastor continued to emphasize the fact that **nothing** ever catches God by surprise, that He has a plan for our lives, even if it includes something as earth-shattering as a pregnant teenager. It is difficult for any parent to go through this kind of shock without some damage, and inside, we were really hurting.

Numb and Shocked

On Sunday afternoon, Kenneth met alone with Patrick and his father. The Freeman family were also just learning the news of the pregnancy, and they were as shocked as we. They were willing to agree with whatever decision Jennifer and Patrick made about their child and their future. It was unanimous that abortion was not a consideration (*"Two wrongs do not make a right"*) ... and I think Patrick was very relieved when we did not demand he marry our daughter. His own mother especially felt that Patrick did not even know if he truly loved Jennifer.

So now there were only two options: either give up the baby for adoption ... or Jennifer would keep the baby and raise him with Patrick's help.

When the family doctor verified Jennifer's pregnancy on the following Monday, estimating she was about twelve weeks pregnant, he too pointed out her various options ... but also encouraged her to not make any decisions quickly. For the next few weeks, it seemed like we were in a weird limbo, and I honestly feared she might opt for the adoption choice. Eventually, she and Patrick chose to keep the baby and try to raise him together as best they could, despite their unpredictable relationship.

God Shows Up Again

As we cautiously shared this devastating news with our extended family and friends, there was much grief and dismay. At one point, my brother-in-law accosted Patrick at our home, and I had to intervene, insisting this young man was the father of my grandchild and should be left alone. It was very difficult telling my widowed father and Kenneth's elderly parents, but we also began experiencing more of God's grace as everyone unconditionally loved Jennifer ... and now were discovering they would need to learn to love Patrick too. It was such a surreal time.

Blindly, hurting so badly, Kenneth and I tried to find our way through this shocking change in our world. Ray and Jo McLeod, close friends of ours, with two daughters of their own, listened sympathetically and lovingly, simply supporting us as friends. They did not offer advice – they just listened ... and never wavered in loving us. Not one of our circle of family and friends criticized or condemned us. I don't know how we would have survived those first weeks without such unconditional, freely given acceptance and care from friends like these.

A week or two after Jennifer's announcement, my sister Judy took me to meet a friend of hers, Linda Knight, who was co-pastoring with her husband a church in Monroe, Washington. Linda also had a very accurate prophetic ministry gift, and Judy believed she could strengthen me in my deep sorrow and lift my bleak outlook on the future.

Linda prayed for me, and God began to speak through her ... and she revealed three very significant things. Through the gift of prophesy, she said, "This child is going to be the salvation of his father and his whole family. This child is going to be a mighty evangelist, and he will win many souls to Christ." That little spark of hope began to brighten even more. I was also astonished to realize that Linda had also identified the gender of the unborn baby: "it" was a "he!"

Another Surprise

A month or so after Jennifer's devastating announcement, one Sunday morning at church Alexander walked to the front and made a public declaration to everyone, which completely surprised Kenneth and me. Having previously discussed this with our pastor, Alexander announced he was choosing to remain a virgin until his wedding day. He stated he was not going to engage in "typical teen dating," but choosing to keep temptation at bay by being only in group scenarios, keeping any physical contact to hand-holding only, and maintaining friendships that never progressed into physical intimacy.

Alexander was true to his commitment: on his wedding day in July 2002, both Alexander and his lovely bride Cherry were virgins. Today they have three lovely children.

Chapter 5: **Our Grandchild's Father**

The relationship Kenneth and I had known with Patrick was merely casual, just a smiling welcome when he came to our home to pick up our daughter for some high school event. Now it changed. Now we had to begin to *see* this young man – although not as the husband of our daughter – as the father of our grandchild. I can't say we were suddenly loving friends ... but we were all made the effort to know each other better, and to respect each other.

While we all live in the same small town (population about 6,000), we really didn't know his family. We were churchgoers, they were not. I remember someone at a high school music concert identifying to me Patrick's father Larry Freeman ... and it turned out Patrick's mother Yvonne was also a client of my hairdresser. His parents had divorced when he was a child, and Patrick, his older sister Tricia and younger brother Chris had been blended into a new family when Larry married Penny, who already had a young daughter Tammy. The Freemans were known as a good, solid family around our little town, but we simply were not acquainted with them.

A Black Hole

One thing about Patrick disturbed me, and that was my "spiritual" perception of him. From the first time I met him, I felt like he was a "walking black hole" – that somewhere deep inside he was broken, although I did not know of any particular reason. When I would look into his handsome, intelligent face and tried to sense his spirit through his eyes, he seemed lifeless, closed, dead.

Several years later, I finally heard the story. When Patrick was 12 or 13 years old, he was forcibly kidnapped from his parents' home and held hostage by a man who physically and sexually abused him. Thankfully, he was rescued within 24 hours, and eventually the abductor was sent to prison. At his parents' insistence, Patrick was given court-ordered counseling, but it had not been very effective, and he subsequently refused any further counseling or emotional therapy. Deep inside, he shut down – away from caring family, away from concerned friends ... and away from God. He didn't believe anyone could "fix" him, and he simply chose to keep that injured part of himself shut away.

Unwillingly, Patrick became an integral part of the life of our family. During her pregnancy, he often spent time with Jennifer at our home, and I was so saddened when I would see them sitting together watching TV, and realized they – as parents of this coming child – should have been sharing the joy and wonder of this little life they had created. Instead, they would sit together (chastely) for a while, then he would go to his home and Jennifer would go alone to her bed to sleep. How well I recalled cuddling in bed with my husband when I was pregnant with Jennifer, having him feel her kicking and rolling in my belly! It was so sad to me they could not experience this wonderful bonding because they were not married ... and not even happy they were pregnant.

"It Happens All the Time"

As summer turned toward autumn, Jennifer entered her senior year of high school. Kenneth and I went to see the school counselor to inform the school that Jennifer was pregnant, asking what the general guidelines would be for "this situation." We should not have been surprised to learn most of the school already knew of her condition, but we were stunned to realize they were completely nonchalant – it was simply something that happened all the time. As far as they were concerned, as long as her health permitted, she could continue with her normal studies. When her delivery date arrived, she could take as much time off school as she needed. They could see no problem with her graduating with her class in June 1993.

Jennifer was not without personal disappointments. The first was when she was dismissed from the Cheerleading Squad. This was a huge loss to her because she really excelled as a cheerleader, and this should have been her shining year. However, being the top of the "human pyramid" was not safe for a pregnant girl, and she had to leave her team of girlfriends who had been cheerleading together for many years. Compared to her pending responsibility for a new human life, Kenneth and I thought her reaction was rather trivial, but in retrospect, it was probably her **last** immature response. From that point forward, Jennifer was determined to focus her attention and energy on her child, to become the very best mother she could.

Jennifer's friends were entirely supportive of her predicament, and of her decision to keep the baby. A couple of male friends even offered to marry her on the spot! I do not know if any of her close friends ever snubbed or disparaged her at all. It is likely none of them were very knowledgeable about the consequences of being a single teenage mother – for instance, shortly after learning of Jennifer's pregnancy, they took her on a river-rafting trip where she became badly (and potentially dangerously) sunburned – but it seems they closed ranks around her rather than kicking her out.

When Kenneth and I had offered to resign from any leadership at our church – which was declined – it was very sweet how our family and friends surrounded us with love and support. This was very kind of them ... but privately, I didn't think we deserved it. I believe this was the first true representation of the shame in which I was becoming engulfed.

Early Impressions

During her regular prenatal visits, Jennifer was scheduled for an ultrasound examination at around 20 weeks.

Patrick took her for the test, and Kenneth and I agreed to meet them at the clinic. We arrived a little later than intended, and the technician was just finishing the exam. I asked for one more quick look at our grandchild ... and when she maneuvered the wand over Jennifer's belly, suddenly we saw two perfect little feet, then a pair of skinny legs, then an unmistakable view of male genitalia!

I clapped my hand over my mouth because I knew Jennifer was hoping for a daughter. I glanced at Patrick, and he was grinning. He told her the baby was a boy, but she stubbornly refused to believe it for the entire pregnancy. (Later that day, I bought the cutest little "tuxedo" pajamas for my grandson to wear someday ... but I didn't make a big deal of it to Jennifer.)

As her pregnancy progressed, she was healthy but did not gain much weight. She refused to wear anything remotely resembling typical maternity clothes, instead choosing to disguise her growing belly with baggy shirts and large sweaters. When we sat for portraits with our extended family, Jennifer stood on the back row, wearing a ruffled dress of mine that completely hid her pregnancy.

On another occasion, when our family attended a church Christmas celebration less than a month before her due-date, we met a longtime friend, Michaela, whom we hadn't seen in several years. Michaela had been our kids' babysitter; now she was a practicing nurse – but even as a medical professional, she did not recognize Jennifer's pregnancy – and she said she thought our daughter looked fantastic and healthy.

Jennifer continued attending school, and her friends continued being completely solicitous of her. Everything about her senior year of high school seemed normal ... except she was 16 and pregnant (and couldn't be a cheerleader anymore). She was as popular as ever, was voted Prom Queen of the Class of 1993, and no one (to my knowledge) ever criticized or condemned her. I can't say how Jennifer felt about this, but perhaps I was absorbing into myself the sense of guilt and shame exhibited I never saw anywhere else. Our society had become immune to sexual sins.

Perhaps because Jennifer was generally disguising her pregnancy and exhibiting a nonchalant attitude about it, this led to me also unconsciously disguising it. I could have told Michaela at the Christmas program that our daughter was pregnant ... but I did not. I did not generally share this news with casual friends or acquaintances. At the time, I don't think I even realized what my feelings were – other than a protectiveness toward my daughter ... and a growing desire to meet my grandchild.

Chapter 6: **Moment of Truth**

Jennifer's due-date was estimated for late January 1993. One Monday, January 11th, Patrick took Jennifer shopping in nearby Bellingham. During the afternoon, she ate Mexican food which she said did not agree with her; she complained her stomach was hurting, and eventually vomited her lunch. (The following Saturday, Patrick and Jennifer had been scheduled to attend a one-day "new parenting" class at the hospital, so neither were particularly aware how to recognize the signs of early labor pains.) They continued shopping, and since it was about two weeks before her due-date, no one else recognized the signs of labor either.

Patrick brought Jennifer home in the early evening, and she continued to complain of a stomachache. It had been an unusually cold winter in our part of Washington State, and that day Kenneth was involved in an icy skid which landed his car in the ditch, so when Jennifer said she wasn't feeling well, he wasn't very sympathetic and told her to "just sleep it off."

I sensed something different. Because I have always had such an interest in childbirth and the wonder of new life, I had long ago taken unofficial training in midwifery. I observed Jennifer carefully, and after a short time of tracking that her "stomach pains" had such regular intervals, I suggested she might be in labor, and we should meet her doctor at the hospital. Although everyone thought it was all a "false alarm," later that evening I drove Jennifer to the hospital, and Patrick soon met us there.

Jennifer's regular doctor had been scheduled to be away at a medical seminar, but the substituting doctor greeted us at the maternity ward. She examined Jennifer, and – to our surprise – said she was about 3 centimeters dilated. Jennifer was admitted as a patient in active labor. By now, Jennifer complained the pain was too much, so they gave her nitrous oxide to breathe in through a mask. Uneasily, Patrick and I settled in with Jennifer in her hospital room, and waited. For Patrick, I expect it was a very strange time – especially since they had not yet taken their parenting class!

"All of a Sudden ..."

After about two hours of labor in the hospital, Jennifer stated she needed to use the toilet. While Patrick was sort of dozing in the corner of the room, the attending nurse and I helped Jennifer get to her feet, and walked her (and the IV stand) to the washroom, waited while she urinated, then helped her shuffle back to the bed. At that point, the nurse suggested another quick pelvic exam would be a good idea. Jennifer climbed back on the bed, the nurse lifted the hospital gown ... and we could both see the baby's head crowning!

"Wash your hands, put on these paper gowns, put on these gloves!" the nurse quickly instructed Patrick and me. "I'm going to call for her doctor." Patrick and I were both a little dumbfounded, I think, because neither of us moved at first. The nurse ran to the main nursing station and paged Jennifer's doctor-on-call. (We did not know then the doctor was in the hospital's cafeteria, but her pager's batteries had died; therefore she did not get the message.) Then the nurse hit this big red alarm button that signaled an impending birth, which I suppose put other attendants on alert. She ran back into Jennifer's room, hastily pulling on her first glove.

I took another look between my daughter's legs, pushed up the sleeves of my sweater, and – with my not-so-sterile, ungloved hands – reached down and grasped the baby's head, which had fully emerged from her body. He was coming out quite quickly, rotating in that way a baby's body does during a normal birth ... but he was not breathing. With one hand gloved and the other not, the nurse suctioned out mucous from the baby's mouth and nose, while I continued gently guiding the still-emerging body. I watched in awe as he took his first breath, and this lovely pink color spread over his slippery body. This was one of the most glorious experiences of my entire life: delivering my own grandson!

With the last little push, the baby was fully born, and it was Patrick who exclaimed, "It's a boy!" While the nurse was cleaning and wrapping the baby, the doctor finally arrived. She offered for Patrick to cut the umbilical cord, but he declined. The doctor then delivered the placenta.

It was early in the morning on Tuesday, January 12, 1993. My precious daughter Jennifer was a mother at age 17, Patrick was a father at age 19, and I was a grandmother at age 39.

The Amazed Look of Wonder and Love

The nurse snuggled the baby in a blanket and laid him in the warming bassinet waiting nearby. I tiptoed over to look at him. The doctor called over her shoulder, "It's okay if you want to pick up the baby." I tenderly lifted my grandson in my arms and carried him to his mother. Jennifer said she was exhausted and declined to hold him quite yet. I then offered him to his father, and Patrick uncertainly took him in his arms ... and this amazed look of wonder and love which passed over his face is a moment I will remember forever.

One thing about being only 17 and having your first baby: it was very easy. The young body is so limber, the muscles have not stiffened with age, and all the parts work well. All together, Jennifer had about 6 hours of labor, the last two being the most intense, and the actual delivery required such minor pushing because the baby seemed so eager to come into the world.

Quickly, I phoned Kenneth and Alexander, asleep at home. They had expected we would call them to come up if or when the birth was near ... they were both a bit disappointed everything had happened so quickly without them! They dressed and came to the hospital right away, as did Patrick's mother Yvonne; later his father Larry and stepmother Penny arrived. Later in the day, my father and other family members trickled in, and more of Patrick's family, and then the parade of Jennifer's and Patrick's friends as everyone welcomed Kristian Michael Alexander Halsey into the world.

(Please note we counseled Jennifer to legally give Kristian her maiden surname, although officially naming Patrick as the father on the birth certificate. It was a decision upon which they both agreed.)

Chapter 7: **A Baby in the House**

A day or two later, Jennifer and Patrick brought their son to our house, and for the next two and a half years, Jennifer and Kristian lived in our home. After a couple of weeks of resting and acclimating to motherhood, Jennifer returned to classes at high school. In June 1993, she graduated with honors.

We loved having Kristian under our roof! He was such a perfect baby: sweet-tempered, healthy, active, and very intelligent. By the age of 18-months, he was quite capable of deliberately selecting the music CD of his choice, inserting the disc, advancing to the track he wanted to hear, and pushing the Play button with glee. Then he would bounce and dance to the music, clapping his hands and crowing with baby-song. In his baby language, he called all music "mee-gock."

It became an anticipated early morning ritual for Kenneth and I to hear his little pajamas-clad feet padding on the floor as he would walk into our bedroom and climb into our bed. Alexander became a combination of uncle and brother to Kristian, and to this day, he is simply known as "Uncle" to our grandchildren. We have countless photos and videos of our family at play with baby Kristian, who was such a precious addition to our family. Everyone loved this little boy!

Another Prophecy Fulfilled

Very soon, the second of Linda Knight's three prophecies (the first being identifying his gender) began to unfold. When Kristian was about 6 weeks old, Jennifer brought him to our home-church, Destiny Christian Church in Bellingham, to have him dedicated to Christ. All the extended families were there: my widower father ... my brothers and sisters and their families ... Patrick's father and his wife ... his mother ... his sister and her husband, with their infant daughter – and our church-family surrounding us with love and acceptance as the pastor performed this simple act of dedication.

During the service, Patrick's stepmother Penny was moved to tears as God began speaking deeply in her heart. She had attended church off-and-on for years, but within the next few Sundays, she was so drawn to the love of God that she made a deep commitment to Jesus Christ. When Larry realized the impact on Penny's life, he too was drawn back to a real and strong relationship with Jesus Christ. Soon both Penny and Larry were regulars at Destiny Christian Church, with Larry often operating the sound-board and helping with ushering, and Penny singing with the worship team. Kenneth and I became good friends with Larry and Penny, and we all rejoiced in our mutual grandson. Patrick's sister Tricia and her husband Brett also renewed their dedication to the Family of God, and began attending another church, along with their infant daughter Kelsey (just months older than Kristian).

At this time, Patrick's mother Yvonne was struggling as an alcoholic divorcee. A few years after Kristian was born, she met and married Bill Carson, also an alcoholic. They began attending Cornwall Church in Bellingham, getting involved with their recovery meetings, and eventually attending a 12-step program together. When they both became stalwart Christians, it became imperative for Yvonne to see all her family saved. Yvonne and I developed a good friendship, and often prayed together for the salvation of her two sons Patrick and Chris.

For many years, Patrick's extended family was the target of much prayer for their salvation. However, I often rejoiced in knowing that because Jennifer brought Kristian into the Family of God through his dedication (which we realize does not substitute for his own personal salvation experience), many of Patrick's family had their walks with God restored as well.

Truly Kristian was a catalyst to change hearts.

Shattered Dreams

After graduating from high school, Jennifer had planned to further her education at college and eventually pursue a career. After a few months at the local university, she realized the care of her little son was more important to her, so she dropped out of college. She took a job at a local retail business so she could maximize spending time with Kristian. When she was working, I was delighted to provide child-care for this little boy whom I loved so passionately.

Although her job was nothing like the career plans she had held, she really excelled in it, and within a short time was given promotion after promotion. By the time Kristian was two-and-a-half, she determined she was making enough income – along with regular financial support from Patrick – to independently support themselves. She found a nearby apartment, and with her roommate Christy Thompson – a close high school friend who was also an unwed mother – and the two young women and their two little boys set up house together. It was a very sad day for us when Jennifer and Kristian moved out of our home, but we also understood her quest for independence ... and we were very relieved that they had not moved very far away.

A Volatile Relationship

I wish I could say Jennifer and Patrick were equally wonderful together. They felt their way carefully through the trials of parenting, and rarely had disagreements over Kristian or his care – but as a woman and a man, their relationship was heading toward disaster. They fought constantly over personal issues ... yet it was equally apparent they loved each other deeply. The stress of teenage parenting is enormous and they managed, but interpersonally they did not fare well at all.

Patrick cared deeply about his son. He visited our home

regularly, and took Kristian to his home often. The entire Freeman family simply absorbed Jennifer and Kristian into their hearts, so pressure was not coming from divided households. It was the same problem we had seen during their dating years: a conflict of personalities, with both being assertive, neither wanting to compromise. I am quite sure they were very glad they had not chosen the marriage option.

Over several years, their difficult personal relationship was strained, finally to a very real breaking point.

Chapter 8: **Acting Out the Lie**

There was this darkness, this sadness, this pain of shame that continued to gnaw inside me. As supportive as we were of Jennifer and her son – and although her peers and our society seemed oblivious to the shame of an unwed teenage mother – I continued to struggle with a sense of "trying to downplay the shame." It finally reached a critical moment in 1994, just over a year after Kristian's birth.

At Christmas 1993 – about a month before Kristian's first birthday (while Jennifer still lived at home) – Kenneth, Jennifer, Alexander, Kristian, and I had posed for a family portrait. There we all were, smiling for the camera – and Kristian was especially adorable with his wide-mouth grin showing off his shiny new teeth – the picture of a happy family. Then in the spring of 1994, Kenneth and I accompanied my father Rev. Don Gossett on another ministry-trip to Australia. In my purse I carried a little pocket-size version of that Christmas family portrait. We missed our daughter, son and grandson intensely, and I often looked at this little picture for comfort.

We met wonderful Australian people, especially at various churches where my father ministered, and they often asked if we had any pictures of our family ... and I would pull out this little photo of the five of us. More often than not, the comment would be something like, "Oh, you have a late-in-life baby! How wonderful!" Most people assumed Kristian was our son, not our grandson ... and so deep was the shame entrenched in my heart that I simply never told them the truth. As much as we loved Kristian for the innocent, wonderful child he was, I quite honestly was ashamed that our daughter's sin of illicit sex and a birth out of wedlock was the evidence. Our beautiful grandson was, in truth, illegitimate, or more harshly, a bastard.

I never once blamed Kristian for his parents' sin. He was not the reason for the shame – it was completely *their* sinful behavior and the consequences they had to endure that broke my heart and made me vulnerable to ongoing sorrow.

The realization finally came that I had been acting out a lie for a long time. Perhaps evidenced by that conversation with Michaela at the Christmas program (when I did not explain Jennifer was pregnant), I was overwhelmed by shame and did not speak the truth. Then, after Kristian was born, the times I had him in my care, especially in public, I never disabused anyone from thinking he was my son. For those who knew the truth about Jennifer and Patrick, it was somewhat of a relief to not have to act the lie ... but if people did not know, neither did I correct their misconceptions.

My Day of Reckoning

While we were in Australia, God "called me into His Office," sat me down in His Chair, and began to deal with my heart. With amazing clarity, He brought back those sermons I had heard Dave Anderson preach a few years before: that when His very own Son Jesus Christ hung on the cross at Golgotha, He took into Himself *all* the sin and *all* the shame that plagues Mankind ... including all the shame with which I was struggling. Just as much as He had forgiven Jennifer and Patrick for their sin, so had He taken all the shame I felt, and forgave that too.

He instructed me that once I repented and gave up the sense of shame to Him, "nailing it to the cross," He could then walk victoriously into my life and totally defeat the enemy who had been consistently robbing me of joy:

God disarmed the principalities and powers that were ranged against us, and made a bold display and public example of them, triumphing over them.

God was calling me to join in His celebration parade, crucifying the very shame with which the enemy had tried to devour and destroy me. Shame does not come from God – it comes from he who is God's greatest enemy. In the Garden of Eden, it was not God Who made Adam and Eve feel ashamed of their nakedness – that was the byproduct of their sin. How this simple truth evaded me, I do not know – but I *did* know I so wanted to be freed from the heaviness of shame that had begun that long, long night in June 1992.

I was trying so hard to be a "perfect" Christian mother and grandmother, I had not realized how effectively Satan had infiltrated my life. He took advantage of the deep wound which shook and unsettled my spiritual and emotional foundations; he took advantage of the break in my heart to slip in a subtle agent that would grow and grow my shame into another sin: untruthfulness. I could not deny the fact that our beloved daughter had become a statistic and her life was forever changed ... but God had more for us!

This is a fundamental truth I really struggled to believe. In my life, God knew there would come challenges, heartbreak, disappointments, hurts, crushing blows – so He has also already prepared His healing and comfort for me:

No temptation has overtaken you except such as is common to Man; but God is faithful, Who will not allow you to be tempted beyond what you are able, but with the temptation will also make the way of escape, that you may be able to bear it.

1 Corinthians 10:13

The *"temptation that overtook me"* was not my own sin, but my **response** to that sin was my own. In a way, I had lost faith in God ... but He was gracious to bring me to my knees, performing necessary surgery on my pain and shame, accepting my repentance, and lifting me up as a whole person:

But we have this treasure in earthen vessels, that the excellence of the power may be of God and not of us. We are hard pressed on every side yet not crushed, we are perplexed but not in despair; persecuted but not forsaken, struck down but not destroyed; always carrying about in the body the dying of our Lord Jesus, that the life of Jesus also may be manifested in our body.

2 Corinthians 4:7-10

Becoming Shame-Free

As I began to process the healing I so desperately needed, this great weight began to slowly lift out of my heart. I cannot say I was instantaneously delivered from shame, but I certainly began a never-turning-back passage away from it. It was not my own understanding or ability that fueled my path to wholeness – it was *"the excellence of the power of God"* that brought me out of sorrow and shame.

When we returned from Australia, I sought my pastor Dr. Kim Ryan for further ministry. At a "ministry time" (an intense prayer meeting, which included two women known as powerful prayer-warriors), I began to lay out all the pain and sorrow I felt, and my shock and dismay over Jennifer's choices and the consequences. I confessed my shame and lack of honesty ... and then was surrounded by their tangible love as the healing of God began to flow. I able to truly exclaim: *"I was hard pressed but not crushed, perplexed but not in despair; persecuted but not forsaken, struck down but not destroyed! I am ready to march with Christ Jesus in His victory parade, reminding Satan that his sticky weight of shame is broken forever in my life! I am shame-free!"* It was an enormous relief.

Our Pure Daughter Restored

Equally important to my acceptance of Christ's forgiveness for my shame and its destructive work in my heart, was our daughter's repentance and her acceptance of God's forgiveness for her sin of fornication. The Bible says it *is* possible to have your wrongs turned around, to have your heart re-made into its original pure state:

"Come now, let's settle this," says the Lord. "Though your sins are like scarlet, I will make them as white as snow. Though they are red like crimson, I will make them as white as wool."

Isaiah 1:18; New Living Translation

He does not punish us for all our sins; He does not deal harshly with us, as we deserve. For His unfailing love toward those who fear Him is as great as the heights of the heavens above the earth. He has removed our sins as far from us as the east is from the west. The Lord is like a Father to His children, tender and compassionate to those who fear Him.

Psalm 103:10-18; NLT

"Then I will forget about their sins and no longer remember their evil deeds." When sins are forgiven, there is no more need to offer sacrifices.

Hebrews 10:17-18; Contemporary English Version

Because of the sacrifice of the Messiah, His blood poured out on the altar of the cross, we're a free people – free of penalties and punishments chalked up by all our misdeeds. And not just barely free, either – abundantly free! He thought of everything, provided for everything we could possibly need, letting us in on the plans He took such delight in making. He set it all out before us in Christ, a long-range plan in which everything would be brought together and summed up in Him, everything in deepest Heaven, everything on Planet Earth.

Ephesians 1:7-10; the Message

Once again I was able to view my daughter with the same unconditional love which overwhelmed my heart on that day when she was born, a pure and precious child.

Chapter 9: **"Forgiven and Set Free"**

For too many years I had been living in some kind of "ivory tower," where I believed that all Christians were good people who tried diligently to obey all the commands and promises of the Bible, and if they succeeded, nothing "bad" would ever happen to them. If something bad *did* happen, it was "an attack of the enemy" and would be overcome by hanging tightly to their faith in God.

I did not focus on the fact that a very real and important part of our Christian walk *includes* facing enormous challenges, great difficulties, huge disappointments, crushing tragedies, sorrows and loss. I was one of those people who gloss over reading about all the Christian martyrs ... and I certainly did not fully understand the teachings of both Jesus Christ and Paul the Apostle:

In this world **you will have tribulation;** *but be of good cheer, for I have overcome the world.*

John 16:33 (emphasis added)

Rejoice in the hope of the glory of God. ... We also glory in tribulation, knowing that tribulation produces perseverance, and perseverance produces character, and character produces hope.

Roman 5:2-4

I thought I knew these Scriptures backward and forward, but I did not grasp that Jesus was specifically telling me to *expect* calamity to invade my life, or that Paul was instructing us how to get through *inevitable* problems. It doesn't get a lot clearer than that, but honestly, I was naive. I knew many Bible verses, but wasn't very good at applying those *"you will have problems"* parts to myself. Now I know I probably would not have survived without some of the precious promises that sustained me during my "shame-filled" zone:

Be strong and of good courage, do not fear nor be afraid of them, for the Lord your God, He is the One Who goes before you. He will not leave you or forsake you.

Deuteronomy 31:6; also see Joshua 1:5 and Hebrews 13:5

Blessed be the God and Father of our Lord Jesus Christ, the Father of mercies and God of all comfort, Who comforts us in all our tribulation, that we may be able to comfort those who are in any trouble with the comfort with which we ourselves are comforted by God. For as the sufferings of Christ abound in us, so our consolation also abounds through Christ.

Now if we are afflicted, it is for your consolation and salvation, which is effective for enduring the same sufferings which we also suffer. Or if we are comforted, it is for your consolation and salvation. And our hope for you is steadfast, because we know that as you are partakers of the sufferings, so also you will partake of the consolation.

2 Corinthians 1:3-7

This was the beginning of a new and very important era in my life, where I began trusting God to take us *through* our challenges. It is not that I felt like He had ever abandoned us, but I had become deluded by the shame I felt inside, so I had stopped trusting Him ... for a while. It was like He began to teach me all again from scratch, and I began to absorb His comforting, restoring Word like a sponge.

The incredible love I have always felt for our daughter was renewed – not that I ever stopped loving her, but my love had become tainted by my shame, and now God cleaned it up and restored it to an even greater degree. The respect and fondness I felt for Patrick was increased – not that I ever doubted his devotion for Kristian (and even, in a convoluted way, for Jennifer), but I no longer looked at him through the film of my pain ... and I was motivated to pray even more fervently for his salvation. The joy I took in Kristian was magnified because I could accept him so much more as God's true gift, even one which came through shocking circumstances. It's not that I became some kind of super-grandmother – it's just once I was set free from shame, I was so strengthened in Christ that I was a better person all around.

God Is Never Surprised

To our astonishment, once Kenneth and I began to be transparent about our daughter and her illegitimate son, in the Christian community we found all sorts of parents who were struggling with the very same thing we had! Maybe we're the oblivious sorts, but we honestly didn't realize there were so many other parents – even in the so-called "holy" Body of Christ! – whose children were illicitly sexually active and who were suffering the consequences. We discovered we most were certainly not alone in this – there were dozens of hurting Christian parents (and even more outside the Church) dealing with these very same problems.

We were asked to counsel with fathers and mothers who sons and daughters were in trouble, and were amazed when we found honest, helpful answers bubbling out of our hearts:

The Father of mercies and God of all comfort, **Who comforts us in our tribulation,** *that we may be able to comfort those who are in any trouble with the comfort with which we ourselves are comforted by God.*

2 Corinthians 1:3-4 (emphasis added)

We were able to help bring peace and comfort to other parents just like us, and I believe they could receive it more readily because they knew we were not just talking theory – we were sharing out of our own experience. It was especially common to hear about the shame these parents felt, and how difficult it was for them to continue to trust God.

Perhaps the first and most important thing we learned

was **God was not surprised by this.** God is never caught unaware or surprised by anything that happens in our lives – for even the trials are part of His plan for us:

Beloved, do not think it strange concerning the fiery trial which is to try you, as though some strange thing happened to you; but rejoice to the extent that you partake of Christ's sufferings, that when His glory is revealed, you may also be glad with exceeding joy.

1 Peter 4:12-13

In this you greatly rejoice, though now for a little while, if need be, you have been grieved by various trials, that the genuineness of your faith – being much ore precious than gold that perishes though it is tested by fire – may be found to praise, honor and glory at the revelation of Jesus Christ.

1 Peter 1:6-7

While those verses refer to our faith as being tested, I view my grandson Kristian as *"being more precious than gold"* and the pride Kenneth and I have in our daughter's accomplishments fill us *"with exceeding joy."* This *"fiery trial"* has been worth it.

We've talked with *many* other parents facing crisis pregnancies, and those who seem to have survived them best have resoundingly echoed the importance of seeking help, of learning to trust God, of leaning on your friends and family, of running *to* the church-family instead of running away in denial and hiding. You might be surprised to learn the Church does not condemn you, they do not judge your pregnant child, and they are willing to share your heavy burden. That's the way God planned it.

Giving Back

I firmly believe God *never* puts His children through any trial or difficulty – always walking *with* us through the test – that He does not expect us to turn around and help somebody else get through that same (or similar) problem:

For everyone to whom much is given, from him much will be required; and to whom much has been committed, of him they will ask the more.

Luke 12:48

What a wonderful God we have – He is the Father of our Lord Jesus Christ, the Source of every mercy, and the One Who so wonderfully comforts and strengthens us in our hardships and trials. And why does He do this? So that when others are in trouble, needing our sympathy and encouragement, we can pass on to them this same help and comfort God has given us.

2 Corinthians 1:3-4; TLB

We are to be Christlike ... that is, "like Christ." Even the Son of God did not waltz through life problem-free – in fact, the very trials He endured had purpose! If He had not become human, we would not have been able to comprehend His limitless compassion and love for us:

(Jesus Christ) was in the world, and the world was made through Him, and the world did not know Him. But as many as received Him, to them He gave the right to become the children of God, to those who believe in His Name; who were born – not of blood, nor of the will of the flesh – but of God. And the Word became flesh and dwelt among us, and we beheld His glory.

John 1:10-14

For Christ also suffered once for sins, the just for the unjust, that He might bring us to God, being put to death in the flesh but made alive by the Spirit.

1 Peter 3:18

He became *"a little lower than the angels"* (Psalm 8:4; also see Hebrews 2:7, 9) so we could understand that *He* truly understands our lives, the difficulties we endure, the disappointments we experience, the problems we face ... and He has a purpose for them. We may not see it at the time, but because **we can absolutely count on Him walking with us through our problems,** we know He will make a way where there seems to be no way.

There was another Scripture that particularly ministered to me as I climbed out of the abyss of shame:

There is therefore now no condemnation to those who are in Christ Jesus, who do not walk according to the flesh but according to the Spirit. For the law of the Spirit of life in Christ Jesus has made me free from the law of sin and death. For what the Law could not do in that it was weak through the flesh, God did by sending His own Son in the likeness of sinful flesh, on account of sin: **He condemned sin in the flesh.**

Romans 8:1-3; emphasis added

There it was again! Because I was yielding to Christ Jesus, He was able to take away the very pain with which I had suffered for so long, and instead make it into a victorious display of His power at work in me, putting Satan to shame for the shame with which he had slimed me.

Of course, I realize there *are* some parents – even Christians – who must take some share of responsibility for the ease with which their children can be tempted into sin, but still there should be no opportunity for Satan to attack them with shame and undermine their faith in God. Being able to trust in God through all the seasons of our lives (see Ecclesiastes 3:1-8) is a very good start. Recognizing that our enemy will do anything to try to destroy us (see 1 Peter 5:8), we must be on guard against him always (see Ephesians 6:10-19) and completely trust in God, no matter what.

*The Spirit of the Lord God is upon me because the Lord has anointed me to preach good tidings to the poor; He has sent me to heal the brokenhearted, to proclaim liberty to the captives and the opening of the prison to those who are bound; to proclaim the acceptable year of the Lord and the day of vengeance of our God; to comfort al who mourn in Zion, **to*** *give them beauty for ashes, the oil of joy for mourning, the garment of praise for the spirit of heaviness; that they may be called trees of righteousness, the planting of the Lord, that He may be glorified.*

Isaiah 61:1-13; emphasis added

When our teenage daughter became pregnant, we thought our whole world had crumbled under our feet. That was merely the first step into being able to accept God's *"beauty for ashes"* and to better know that He is trustworthy always.

Part Two: **Romans 8:28**

For we are saved by hope; but hope that is seen is not hope, for what a man sees, why does he yet hope for? But if we hope for that we see not, then do we with patience wait for it. Likewise the Spirit Itself makes intercession for us with groaning that cannot be uttered. And He Who searched the heart knows what is in the mind of the Spirit because He makes intercession for the saints according to the will of God.

And we know that all things work together for good to those who love God, to those who are the called according to His purpose.

Romans 8:24-28; emphasis added

Chapter 10: **The Little Evangelist**

In the years which followed the first rendition of this book (1995), we continued to have a wonderful relationship with our daughter and grandson, and a warm connection with Patrick. He was quite different from our family: our idea of a "fun family vacation" is going to Disneyland – his idea is camping in the great outdoors. He would sometimes go to church with us, but it was obvious he was disinterested in anything to do with God.

It was difficult to watch Jennifer and Patrick's frequent clashes, and we tried to shield Kristian from their problems. Patrick was not even remotely a Christian, and he struggled with drinking and partying issues. He dated other women, which often hurt Jennifer's heart tremendously. She remained celibate, although her being a single mother seemed to not be a problem for any of the young men she knew. She had one male friend who asked her several times to marry him, offering to adopt Kristian – whom he greatly loved as well – but Jennifer turned him down repeatedly.

After I went through the catharsis of allowing God to draw out my sense of shame over Jennifer's situation, I cannot say I never struggled with it ever again. There came a day, however, when I realized just how well God had healed my heart.

When Kristian was about four-years-old, one day I took him to his preschool class at Grace Lutheran Church in Blaine. He was such a vivacious child, and we always had much fun together. On this particular winter day, I walked with him into the classroom and was helping him take off his coat in the coatroom. Just outside the coatroom, another mother was dropping off her child, and she was chatting with the preschool teacher. This young mother was a distant relation of Patrick; she was not known for her discretion. I overheard her say, "Well, I see that my cousin's bastard has arrived."

I couldn't believe my ears! Such a harsh, condemning statement to make ... and about an innocent child who was related to her! I don't know if the teacher responded at all, but I suddenly erupted from the coatroom and stared at Patrick's cousin. When she realized I had overheard her judgmental comment, she turned about five shades of red with embarrassment.

There was a moment when I could have punched her in the face for such a nasty word being applied to my beloved grandson – but then I clearly heard Holy Spirit say, "That is technically true. Kristian is the result of an illicit union. He *is* a bastard. He is not to blame ... and in My eyes, he is pure and innocent of any sin." I gave this small-minded woman a rather fake smile, but I proudly took Kristian's hand and walked him into the classroom. Even my "justifiable anger" had been defeated by God's healing grace.

The A-B-C's of Evangelism

In the summer of 2001, eight-year-old Kristian attended Vacation Bible School at Cornwall Park Church of God in Bellingham. Jennifer drove him to the week-long class in the mornings, and Patrick was responsible to pick him up at noon and take him home. The young students of this VBS were engaged in a contest to see which children could learn "The A-B-C's of Evangelism" and win prizes at the end of the week. Kristian was very motivated to win.

Each day when Patrick picked him up, Kristian jumped into the car and began to hammer his father, "Listen, Daddy, I want to win the prize! So help me with my Bible verses: *A – 'For ALL have sinned and fall short of the glory of God'* ... *B –*

'BELIEVE on the Lord Jesus Christ and you shall be saved ... C –
'CONFESS our sins, and He is faithful and just to forgive our sins and
cleanse use from all unrighteousness ..." and so on. Patrick simply
did not stand a chance: day after day, he was being blasted by
his eight-year-old son with the Gospel of Jesus Christ! Despite
his resistance, God's Word was making its way into his heart.

Later that summer of 2001, the whole Freeman clan
(including Jennifer and Kristian) went camping at Lake
Chelan; this was a regular family event. Jennifer invited her
high school friend Michelle McDonald to join them, and she
drove in her own car over the mountains to eastern
Washington. Something pivotal happened there ... something
life-changing.

Literally on the Mountaintop

From what we have been told, it appears Jennifer and
Patrick engaged in a ferocious argument, and the whole
Freeman family heard it. We never learned *what* it was about,
but the next thing we knew Jennifer was calling her father and
me from her mobile phone, and with angry tears evident in her
voice, she stormed, "I've had it! I never want to see Patrick
Freeman again! I never want to have anything to do with him,
ever! When he wants to see Kristian, he will have to arrange it
through you. He'll have to come to your house to pick him up,
and he will have to bring him back to you. I never want to see
him again!"

Jennifer, Kristian and Michelle were already driving
home when she blazed this furious statement on the phone; they
had left Lake Chelan after being there only one night. Kenneth
and I looked at each other with amazement and concern. Their
relationship had been up and down, but they had weathered
storms before. This sounded serious.

What happened next was related by Patrick's
stepmother Penny. Evidently shortly after Jennifer left Lake

Chelan, Patrick packed up his camping gear and headed out too
– but no one knew where he was going. Penny said she was
very worried about her stepson, and very concerned about this
sudden deterioration of Jennifer's and Patrick's relationship.
All she knew to do was to pray. How the rest of this unfolds
has an almost dreamlike quality.

Patrick drove to Mount Baker in western Washington,
about 50 miles from Blaine. He set up his tent in a wilderness
campsite, intending to be alone. And alone he was for a couple
of days, processing the huge rift that had developed between
him and Jennifer. Finally, he started talking to God:

"God, You see how badly I have messed up. I have been
in control of my life, but I have done a very poor job of it. I
don't know what to do now. Jennifer has cut me off. My
relationship with my son is in danger. I don't know what to do.
I have done such a terrible job of running my own life that I am
giving it up to You. You take over. You take control of my life.
I need Your help."

All those Bible verses of the "A-B-C's of Evangelism"
began to flood through Patrick's brain and into his heart. Then
he knew what he had to do: he prayed the Sinner's Prayer,
repenting of his sins and giving control of his life to Jesus
Christ ... and a huge transformation took place! It was like he
began to shed thick, thick layers of the years of pain from the
effects of his childhood kidnapping and molestation, and was
able to let go of his anger against God. Now he was free to love
and be loved. (Ta da! Linda Knight's third prophesy – that
Kristian would be instrumental in winning his father to
salvation through Jesus Christ – was being fulfilled.)

The next thing he did was pack up his camp and drive
straight to Jennifer's home in Birch Bay. (By this time,
Jennifer – who is very good with her money – owned her own
house, all her furniture and appliances, was driving a new car,
and was debt-free.) She was startled to see Patrick turn up on

her doorstep ... but she let him in. He poured it all out, asking her forgiveness for their so-strained, difficult relationship. Then he asked her to marry him. He loved her with all his now-whole heart, and he wanted to be with her for the rest of their lives. He wanted them to become a complete family.

And Jennifer – who has ever only loved one man in her life – accepted his proposal.

Right-Side Up

When Jennifer told us she was going to marry Patrick Freeman, we were completely astounded. One moment she was raging he had hurt her for the last time and she never wanted to see him again ... and the next (okay, it was several days), she was professing her great love for him and her desire to marry him.

Truthfully, I cannot say I was completely convinced my daughter's world was suddenly turned right-side up again. (In my youth I had "evangelistically dated" boys whom I knew were not Christian, yet sometimes they went through the motions of praying the Sinner's Prayer so I would continue dating them. When I realized what they were doing, I always severed the relationship immediately.) You just cannot fake being a Christian – either Jesus becomes Lord of your life, or He is not.

I asked to speak with Patrick for myself ... and the very first thing I noticed was there was light in his eyes! I previously mentioned that most of my encounters with him made me feel like he was a "walking black-hole," that his eyes always looked dead (except for that one time when he first held his newborn son). Now, as he shared what God had done in his life, this softly glowing light was shining through his eyes. I was literally seeing *"a new creation in Christ"* (see 2 Corinthians 5:17) being made right before my eyes!

Patrick asked Kenneth for permission to marry our

daughter, and he consented. A wedding date was set for April 6, 2002. It was a fabulous turnaround in all our lives.

About a month later, I accompanied my sister Judy Gossett to a women's church conference in Washington, D.C. During one service, the speaker asked all those in the audience who had unsaved loved ones among their family and friends to stand for prayer on their behalf. In the ten years since Patrick Freeman had come into our lives, again and again I had asked for prayer for his salvation. This night, I automatically stood up ... and then suddenly it occurred to me that I no longer had to pray for Patrick's salvation! I sat back down in my seat laughing and crying at the same time. My son-in-law (to-be) had finally come home!

Chapter 11: **Wonders Never Cease**

Filled with wonder, we began to prepare for our daughter's wedding. (Coincidentally, our son also announced his engagement, with plans to marry four months after Jennifer's – talk about "breaking the bank!") Nearly as surreal as that time when we experienced the devastation of Jennifer's pregnancy announcement, now we were experiencing the excitement of planning Jennifer's and Patrick's wedding.

In the spring of 2002, Kristian and I accompanied Jennifer and Patrick to the County Courthouse. While his parents were on the main floor applying for their marriage license, Kristian and I took the elevator up to another department because he wanted to apply to officially change his name from "Kristian Halsey" to "Kristian Freeman." This was very important to him – and made me realize he too understood the sting of being born to unwed parents, and he wanted to be made legitimate in every way. I never knew what kind of problems he might have personally encountered about his unmarried parents, but this was a quite a statement for a 9-year-old boy to make.

(Technically, when the father is acknowledged on the birth certificate, and he accepts responsibility for the care and upbringing of his child, the child is not considered to illegitimate or a bastard.)

For me, there was a bittersweet moment of relinquishing my precious grandson from his unwed parents to his rightful position as the acknowledged son of their soon-to-be marriage. That was likely when the very last vestige of shame evaporated forever.

God's Promises Fulfilled

When we designed their wedding invitation, we included the Scripture reference of Romans 8:28 on the front:

For God causes all things to work together in His timing for good to those who love God, to those who are called according to His purpose (paraphrased).

We never asked for our "perfect" 16-year-old daughter to become pregnant outside of marriage. We never asked for her life to become difficult or her future so uncertain because of her choices, or for her relationship with Patrick to be so volatile. And we could never have asked for such a wonderful grandson to be born into our family! We could never have foreseen how God was going to use that child – even as Linda Knight's prophecies had foretold – to contribute to the salvation of his father and his family. We never wanted those years of anxiety and incompletion for Jennifer and Patrick, and Kristian. But our loving, infinite, caring, knowing Heavenly Father knew what He was doing all along!

God took the ashes of our dreams for our daughter and her future ... and on a lovely, rainy Saturday morning at Cornwall Church in Bellingham, Washington, our grandson stood beside his father and Uncle Chris (his father's best man) at the front of the church and watched his mother come gliding down the aisle on the arm of her father – God restored such beauty! It was a glorious day with many tears of joy, laughter and celebration of what God had done in all their lives.

Within the year, 29-year-old Patrick and 10-year-old Kristian were water-baptized at the same service at Cornwall Church. Shortly after, Chris Freeman finally came to know Jesus as his Savior and Lord, and he is now happily married to Gina, with two sweet children. God's love is never divided – it always multiplies!

Of Cakes and the Icing Thereon

Almost four years later, when Jennifer was 30 and

Patrick 32, they were blessed with another child: Ava Michelle Freeman, who was born on February 3, 2006 (Kristian had just turned 13). This time, it was not such a textbook delivery ... but let's hear Patrick tell this in his own words (as he wrote in an email to family and friends):

Tuesday February 7, 2006 ~ Hello, Family and Friends. We are all doing well and happy to be home. Jen and I went to the hospital Friday afternoon after Jen's contractions started to come about 3 to 4 minutes apart. She was admitted, and given an epidural shortly after. We expected a somewhat long night as Jen's contractions were somewhat close and evenly spaced, but she was only dilated 3 to 4 centimeters. The only complication so far was the baby's heart rate: it tended to fluctuate (lower) when Jen changed position and, surprisingly, whenever the doctor examined her. The doctor at this point (around 4 or 4:30pm) mentioned to us there was a chance that the baby's umbilical cord could be wrapped around her neck, thus causing the fluctuations. He also briefly discussed the slight chance that Jen may need to deliver via Caesarean-section.

The doctor came in again at around 6:30 and examined Jen and the baby, and determined we were still a ways out. We spent the next two and a half hours watching the machine that showed both the baby's heart and also the strength and frequency of Jen's contractions. Baby Ava's heart rate would drop often between contractions; sometimes a bit, sometimes alarmingly low. At about 9:15, Jen's doctor came back to see her. As he examined her, we discussed again the possibility of a C-section if the baby's heart rate didn't stabilize. Almost at that exact time, Ava's heart rate dropped to 55 to 60 beats-per-minute (it should be between 120 and 160). The doctor and nurses in attendance shifted Jen's position several times, trying to get Ava's rate up to within normal. I had watched the doctor and nurses work with Jen all day, and was extremely impressed by their professionalism. Watching them become more and more agitated by Jen and particularly Ava's condition as the minutes ticked by was unnerving, to say the least.

The doctor, after about 2 minutes, made the decision to deliver Ava via C-section, and within another minute, they had moved Jen out of the [labor] room and everyone was gone. It was a surreal moment. The room I was in – which was bustling with activity only a moment ago – was empty except for myself. Not knowing really what else to do or what was going on, I began to pray for Jen and Ava's safety, and for the staff of the hospital. Not more than 50 feet away, my parents, Jen's parents and Kristian heard the "Code Purple in Room 1" announcement over the intercom system, and realizing that they were talking about Jen, began to pray as well. It's interesting now, when I think back about that little bit, maybe 10 to 12 minutes in all, that it seemed to me to be an eternity.

Eventually, someone came in to "suit me up" so I could go into the operating room, and also strangely enough, to sign some consent forms for Jen's C-section – which I'm pretty sure had already occurred. Finally, I got to go in. It seemed to me that every doctor and nurse in the hospital had squeezed into the operating room to make sure that everything went smoothly. There were, by my count, at least 12 to 14 people working to insure Jen and Ava's safety. It was incredible and very touching to see the concern every single one of these people had for my family.

It turns out that everything had gone very smoothly in spite of the previous events of the evening. Ava had gotten her umbilical cord wrapped around her neck not once but twice, and tied it into two different knots. She is apparently quite the acrobat. Jen is quite the patient, and got a laugh or two from everyone in the OR, particularly when she asked if she could get a nose job while she was in there. I walked Ava to the Special Care Nursery, where they gave her a once-over and declared her to be a beautiful, healthy baby (I could have told them that).

We spent a restless Friday and Saturday in the hospital, and I think by Sunday, we were all ready to go home. We can't say enough about the staff at the hospital – they were incredible – but if you're looking to get some rest, you're not going to get it at a hospital! When Jen's doctor came in Sunday morning to check on Jen and Ava, and asked if we would like to go home that day, we were thinking some time that night. In fact, we got home by about 11:00am Sunday morning. We got some good rest yesterday and last night, and are slowly adjusting to having a new member of our family.

Jen and I were talking today about how blessed we feel – not only for God having given us a beautiful, healthy girl – but for all of you who have prayed for and kept us in your thoughts lately. I feel especially blessed for the whole experience of this last weekend. I know that God is always with us, but I could feel Him in that hospital Friday night, as much as I could reach with my left hand and feel my right. I know that His hand was on Ava during that complicated time, and guiding the hands of all those wonderful people in the OR. It truly was an amazing night.

For me, this makes a perfect, awesome ending to this beautiful story. As God continues to bless us with grandchildren, we overflow with joy and gratitude for every sweet little person He brings into our lives. Kenneth and I have so many treasures:

- **Jennifer,** our wonderful daughter, with whom we have walked through the most challenging trial of our lives;

- our priceless son **Alexander,** who continues to be a valiant man of God, serving full-time on the mission-field of India;

- our brilliant grandson **Kristian,** whose life is so precious to us;

- our handsome son-in-law **Patrick,** the most transformed man I know;

- vivacious **Ava,** Jennifer and Patrick's incredible daughter;

- our beautiful daughter-in-law **Cherry,** Alex's sweet India-born wife;

- Alexander and Cherry's beloved children, delightful **Jude** (born October 2005), adorable Aja (born February 2007) and sweet **Hayley** (born February 2009).

Every life is God's gift, and I thank Him for His continual presence throughout my life, *especially* when I did not sense Him. He has made me completely shame-free!

My Last Comment

"I know that God is always with us, but I could feel Him in that hospital Friday night, as much as I could reach with my left hand and feel my right." Those are awesome words which Patrick Freeman wrote ... and even more amazing considering they came from a man who did not know God 17 years before, when he and Jennifer engaged in premarital sex that resulted in pregnancy, when he was not a candidate to marry our daughter because he was an unbeliever.

People think "crisis pregnancy" centers are just about saving unborn children. While that is true, in a sense they really are about *saving lives,* about helping people find God. In 1992, when our beautiful daughter got pregnant, I did not know about the Whatcom County Pregnancy Clinic, but I later learned it had been in business only a year or two then. If only we had known there was a haven all of us could go to help us get through the turmoil of a crisis pregnancy! It's no wonder I have such a strong commitment to purity and abstinence, and have worked with the Clinic to help tell that story to teenagers everywhere.

Not every parent is going to have this "happily ever-after" sort of story to tell. In fact, more broken-hearted parents of pregnant teenage children will wonder, *"How can something good come out of something so awful?"* ... *"When will the shock and pain become less hurtful?"* ... *"What is going to happen to our child, our grandchild, and us?"*

Our shock was because we did not know what Jennifer was doing – our shame came when we realized we would all have to live with these consequences for the rest of our lives.

In truth, most of my sense of shame selfishly came from wondering what people were going to think of Kenneth and me as Jennifer's parents, and less what would be their opinion of our daughter. In retrospect, that was so narcissistic. Maybe it comes from the misguided sense that something as tragic as a pregnant teenage child has never happened to anyone else – that we were alone in totally uncharted territory with this tragedy. But as I noted previously, after we survived this experience, all sorts of grieving parents suddenly showed up, asking for hope.

Here is what I absolutely know: during the height of this crisis in our lives nor in the years that followed, never once did we ever sense God had abandoned us, that we were useless parents, that there was never going to be any relief from this pain, that He had given up on us or Jennifer or Patrick. When I could not sense "hope" anywhere, at least I never lost that sense of His love for me. I held on to His love ... and He guided me through *"the valley of the shadow of shame"* (to paraphrase the Psalmist).

Chapter 12: **Finale**

There is one final memory I'd like to share. About an hour after the drama of Ava's difficult birth, when we (Yvonne and Bill, Kenneth, Kristian, and I) were finally permitted into Jennifer's hospital room, there we found her lying serenely with this tiny, perfect little baby in her arms. As I leaned down to kiss my daughter's cheek, so enjoying the adoring expression on her face, she softly said, "I think I'll keep her." I had to pause and slowly search through my memory banks ... and then I retrieved it.

It was a recollection from thirteen years before. About an hour after Jennifer had given birth to Kristian and was resting quietly, I watched her gazing at her new son. And she whispered, "I think I'll keep him." It was a completely spontaneous expression from her heart, and it totally endeared her to me all over again, reassuring me she was going to be a great mother. To hear her say this again at Ava's birth renewed my love, pride and trust in Jennifer even more.

Today, Patrick works for the City of Blaine; he has custom-built his family a lovely new home in Blaine, only 4 miles from our house. Jennifer is Chief Financial Officer of *Bold Bible Missions,* and a very successful realtor with *Century 21 Bay Properties.* Kristian was voted by acclamation as the Vice President of the Associated Student Body in his junior year at Blaine High School; he maintains a 3.95 GPA, keeps busy with music (guitar, percussion, keyboards), and is a computer genius. Pretty little Ava comes to my house two or three days a week, where she constantly delights her Grammy.

We do not know what paths our lives will take next, but every one of us can hold on tightly and securely to this promise:

No matter what happens to us, God will never leave us, will never abandon us to shame and grief, and is perfectly capable of turning sorrow into joy.

What He has done for us to free us from shame, He can do for you.

A Postscript From Kristian

When my grandmother told me about this book, I was a little worried, but she handled telling this difficult story with accuracy and grace. It is surreal reading about my father and mother, and what they went through because of their choices. I also didn't expect to be written up like some kind of a hero!

Certainly it causes you think about what choices you want to make with your own life, realizing the possible consequences of teenage or premarital sex. I hope this story will help teenagers and their parents if facing an unplanned pregnancy, to know that God never gives up on them and can really help them face their problems with hope.

Recommended Resources

"Mom, Dad ... I'm Pregnant" by Jayne E. Schooler; published 2004 by NavPress (Post Office Box 35001, Colorado Springs, Colorado, 80935, U.S.A.); www.navpress.com

"How to Survive Your Teen's Pregnancy" by Linda Ellen Perry; published 2003 by Chalfont House (Post Office Box 84, Dumfries, Virginia, 22026, U.S.A.); www.chalfonthouse.com

"I'll Hold You in Heaven" by Jack Hayford; published 2003 by Regal Books from Gospel Light (Post Office Box 3875, Ventura, California, 98006, U.S.A.); www.regalbooks.com

The Whatcom County Pregnancy Clinic, 1310 North State Street, Bellingham, Washington, 98225, U.S.A.; 360.671.9057; info@whatcomclinic.com

CareNet; www.care-net.org

About the Author

Jeanne Halsey (born 1953) is a daughter, sister, wife, mother, grandmother ... and a talented writer. Third of five children born to international missionary-evangelist Dr. Don Gossett and (the late) Joyce Gossett, Jeanne naturally inherited her father's "gift of writing" (he has published over 120 books, including the best-selling *"What You Say Is What You Get"* and the ever-popular *"My Never Again List"*). Jeanne was born in Oklahoma ... immigrated to Canada at age 7 ... was educated in British Columbia (Douglas Junior College, the University of British Columbia) ... and has lived in British Columbia, Washington state, Texas, and Colorado. She has traveled internationally extensively.

Former Managing Editor of two internationally distributed monthly Christian magazines, Jeanne is now a freelance writer. She has ghosted and published books for several renowned Christian ministries and contemporary personalities: for her father; Robert Tilton; Marilyn Hickey; Danny Ost; Cliff Self; Benny Hinn; Sarah Bowling; Reinhard Bonnke; Paul Overstreet; U. Gary Charlwood; and many others. She has written for Christian and secular trade magazines, and published several Sports articles about NBA superstar Luke Ridnour for *Sports Spectrum* Magazine. She also publishes an Internet newsletter, *e-Jeanne,* and regularly teaches Creative Writing classes.

Jeanne lives in Blaine, Washington, with her husband (since 1974) **Kenneth Halsey,** a Vice President of Franchise Sales for the *Realogy Corporation;* and their "empty-nest home" includes an American Cocker Spaniel, Maraschino Valentino, and a Chihuahua named Lucia Gracias. Their beautiful daughter **Jennifer** is married to **Patrick Freeman**; they have two children, **Kristian** and **Ava**; and thankfully they live very nearby in Blaine. Their talented son **Alexander** is married to **Cherry Ruth**; they have three children, **Jude, Aja** and **Hayley**; they live halfway around the world, stationed in India as missionary-teachers with *Youth With a Mission.*

Jeanne is an outspoken activist for Christian causes and has stood for public office (she lost). She is past-Chair of the Board of Directors of the *Whatcom County Pregnancy Clinic.* Jeanne and Kenneth are active members of *North County Christ the King Community Church* in Lynden, Washington.

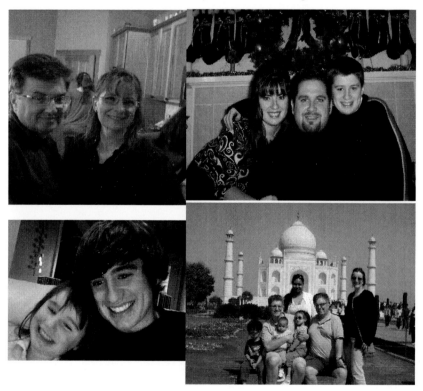

Other Titles by Jeanne Halsey

Nonfiction

Behold the Lamb (an Easter Bible Study)

Three Strikes! (Dealing with Apathy, Ingratitude and Unbelief)

As For Me and My House ("How to Win Your Loved Ones to Christ") with Don Gossett

Born to Conquer with Don Gossett

The Ministry of Angels and Believers with Don Gossett

Protect Yourself In a World of Danger with Don Gossett

Great Transactions of the Power of God for William Canada Shackelford

Don's Daily Devotions with Don Gossett

If Nobody Reaches, Nobody Gets Touched with Don Gossett

The School of Praise with Don Gossett

The School of Blessing with Don Gossett

Win the Lost At Any Cost (The Danny Ost Story) with Harald Bredesen

How to Receive and Keep Your Healing for Robert Tilton

Break the Generation Curse for Marilyn Hickey

Through the Bible for Marilyn Hickey

The Church Alive in Shanghai for Paul Crawford and Bishop Aloysius Lu-xian

Courage: How to Make Things Happen for Cliff Self

Take Your Freedom for Rita Lecours

My Knight in Shining Armor with Linda Knight

The End Times Are Over, So What Are You Afraid Of? with Mike Dearinger and Bob Seymour

What's That You Have In Your Hands?

Solutions for Sarah Bowling

Fearless on the Edge for Sarah Bowling

Mark My Word (year-long devotional) for Reinhard Bonnke

Forever and Ever, Amen for Paul Overstreet

The Legacy of Writing

It's Not About Me for Bryan Duncan

Naked With God

Follow the Yellow Brick Road Workbook with Reba Rambo-McGuire and Judy Gossett

Training the Human Spirit for Rogé Abergel

In Him for Randy Gilbert

Unlimited Potential in Christ for Kim O. Ryan

Falling Out of the Tower

Exit the Dragon: Fierce Faith Meets Modern Medicine

The Mark of the King for Garth McFadden

Fiction

And God Created Theatre

The Ministry of Drama

The Eye-For-An-Eye-Witness News Skits

Messiah! Bright Morning Star Stage Play, with Reba Rambo-McGuire and Dony McGuire, William & Gloria Gaither, and Judy Gossett

Bittersweet (a novel of King David and his first wife Michel)

That Which I Ought to Do (a novel of Paul the Apostle)

Anna the Donkey (a children's Christmas story)

Ya-Ya (a novel)

A Christmas Fantasy for Jude and Ava

An Easter Fantasy for Jude, Ava and Aja

Another Fantasy for Jude, Ava, Aja, and Hayley

The Blue Vial (a children's science-fiction trilogy)